ESSENTIAL GUIDE TO KELOIDS

Comprehensive Insights and Effective Treatments for Scar Management

DR. CASEY LOREN

1

DISCLAIMER

This book's content is only meant to be used for general informative purposes. Although the author has taken great care to ensure the content is accurate and thorough, no warranties or assurances on the information's accuracy, correctness, or reliability are provided. It is recommended that readers employ their own judgment and discretion when applying any material found in this book to their particular situation.

The information in this book is not intended to replace professional advice, nor is the author an expert in any of the subjects covered. It is recommended that readers consult with experienced professionals regarding any particular issues or concerns.

Any name that may be mentioned or referred in this book does not imply endorsement, recommendation, or relationship on the part of the author with any person, entity, good, website, or association. These references are made only for informational purposes and are not meant to be taken as recommendations or endorsements.

The information contained in this book may cause readers to suffer loss or damage, for which the author disclaims all obligation and accountability. The only people accountable for the decisions and actions taken by readers using the information presented are themselves.

Any names, characters, companies, locations, activities, occasions, and incidents referenced in this book are either made up or the result of the author's imagination. Any likeness to real people, living or dead, or to real things is entirely coincidental.

This book's content may change at any time, without prior notice, according to the author.

The onus is on the reader to verify whether there have been any updates or revisions.

The reader accepts the conditions of this disclaimer by reading this book. Please do not read this book or use its contents if you do not agree to these terms.

Table of Contents

CHAPTER 1

COMPREHENDING KELOIDS

Keloids Explained

When scar tissue forms abnormally at the site of a healed skin lesion, it can result in keloids, which are elevated, thickened patches of skin. Keloids do not retract with time and extend beyond the initial incision borders, in contrast to conventional scars. They are regarded as benign (non-cancerous) fibrous growths that can develop after burns, surgical incisions, acne, chickenpox, and even small abrasions.

Background and History

Keloids have been recognized since antiquated medical books. The Greek word "chele," which means "crab's claw," is where the term "keloid" comes from, referring to their protrusion that resembles claws into the surrounding skin. From straightforward observations of aberrant scarring to a more profound comprehension of their pathogenesis, historical accounts have developed. Although hypertrophic scars were once mistakenly associated with keloids, advances in medical science have now identified keloids as a separate disorder.

Distinctions Between Other Scars and Keloids

Although both keloids and hypertrophic scars are forms of excessive scar tissue, they differ in certain ways:

Keloids: Grow over time, do not spontaneously regress, and extend beyond the confines of the initial wound. They are frequently bigger and more noticeable and can appear months after the initial injury.

Hypertrophic Scars: Regress frequently throughout time, remain inside the original wound limits, and may become flatter and less visible in the absence of treatment.

Typical Indications and Features

There are multiple distinguishing characteristics of keloids:

- **Appearance:** Smooth, pink, crimson, or darker-colored skin growths that are elevated and shiny relative to the surrounding skin.

- **Texture:** Texturally springy and firm.

- **Size and Shape:** Range in size from uneven bulk to tiny nodules.

- **Symptoms:** Tenderness, soreness, itching, and perhaps limited mobility if the condition is close to a joint.

Keloids Types

Keloids can be grouped according to where they come from and how they look:

- **Spontaneous Keloids:** Develop often in susceptible persons without a discernible original injury.

- **Post-traumatic Keloids:** Emerge after burns, cuts, or surgical incisions on the skin.

Ear Keloids: Often occur following ear piercings.

- **Acne Keloids:** Develop in reaction to severe lesions of acne.

Who Is at Risk for Keloids?

Certain demographics and conditions are more conducive to the production of keloids:

Genetics: The likelihood of developing keloids is higher in those with a family history of the condition.

Ethnicity: Those with darker skin tones, such as those who identify as African, Hispanic, or South Asian, are more likely to have this condition.

Age: More common in younger people, especially in the 10 to 30 age range.

Gender: Slightly more prevalent among women, maybe as a result of more people getting skin procedures and ear piercings.

How To Form Keloids

Keloid formation's precise method is an excessive reaction to skin injury:

1. **Wound Healing Process:** Normally, collagen is produced by the skin to mend itself. This mechanism becomes dysregulated in keloids.

2. **Overproduction of Collagen:** Fibroblasts, the cells that produce collagen, become hyperactive, which results in an overabundance of collagen deposition.

3. **Inflammatory Response:** Abnormal scar formation is sustained by extended inflammation and growth factor release.

Environmental and Genetic Factors

Keloid growth is influenced by environmental stimuli as well as genetic predisposition:

Genetic Factors: People may be more susceptible to developing keloid formation if they have mutations in genes linked to collagen synthesis and wound healing.

- **Environmental Factors:** Certain forms of skin injuries, recurrent trauma, and skin tension can all raise the risk.

Keloids' Psychological Effects

Keloids have a substantial impact on a person's mental health:

- **Self-Esteem:** Prominent and visible keloids may cause a person to feel self-conscious and less confident.

- **Social Anxiety:** Social disengagement and anxiety can be brought on by a fear of social stigma and unfavorable attention.

- **Depression:** Symptoms of depression may be exacerbated by ongoing discomfort and appearance-related unhappiness.

Untruths Regarding Keloids

There are a few widespread misunderstandings regarding keloids that require explanation:

- **Contagiousness:** Keloids are not communicable and do not transfer from one individual to another.

- **Infectious Origin:** Atypical wound healing, not infections, is the origin of them.

- **Uniform Appearance:** Not all raised scars are keloids, and keloids differ widely in size, shape, and color.

- **Ease of therapy:** Recurrence following therapy is common, and keloids can be difficult to treat.

Comprehending these facets of keloids is essential for accurate diagnosis, treatment, and resolving the worries of individuals impacted by this ailment.

CHAPTER 2
REASONS AND DANGER ELEMENTS

Hereditary Propensity

Actinic keratosis (AK) development is significantly influenced by genetic factors. Atypical kernel formation (AKs) can result from specific genetic abnormalities that heighten vulnerability to UV-induced skin damage. Higher incidences of AK are frequently seen in families with a history of skin malignancies, including squamous cell carcinoma, suggesting a genetic predisposition. Furthermore, because hereditary conditions like xeroderma pigmentosum cannot properly repair UV-induced DNA damage, they significantly increase the risk of acquiring numerous AKs at a young age.

Trauma and Skin Injuries

People who have had repeated trauma or skin injuries may be more susceptible to actinic keratosis. Prolonged physical harm to the skin can lead to structural alterations and localized immunosuppression, which increases the skin's vulnerability to UV radiation's carcinogenic effects. As a result of an extended wound-healing response that encourages aberrant keratinocyte proliferation, AKs can appear in skin regions that are often wounded or abraded.

Keloids and Surgical Procedures

Despite not having a direct connection to actinic keratosis, surgical operations can affect how the skin heals and the generation of keloids, which are scar tissue overgrowths. People who are prone to keloid formation frequently have an overreaction to healing, which can make surgical outcomes more difficult. Although indirect, there is a noteworthy correlation between surgical scars, keloids, and AK, particularly in individuals who need numerous surgical procedures for skin disorders.

Keloid Formation and Acne

Scarring from severe acne can eventually turn into keloids in certain people. Acne's inflammatory nature can set off an overzealous healing process that leads to keloid development and excessive collagen deposition. While keloids do not in and of themselves constitute a risk factor for AK, their presence suggests an elevated inflammatory response to skin injury, which may have implications for understanding how individuals react to UV exposure and the likelihood of developing AKs.

Keloids and Burns

Burns can leave large scars and keloid development, especially if they involve extensive tissue damage. A burn injury requires considerable healing, which may result in an aberrant scar reaction. Although the main issue remains the cosmetic and functional consequences of keloid scars, severe burns, like other forms of trauma, might undermine the skin's integrity, thus raising the likelihood of UV-induced damage and eventual AK formation in the afflicted areas.

Tattoos and Piercings

In those who are vulnerable, intentional skin damage from piercings and tattoos can result in keloid formation. Keloids can result from these operations' recurrent stress and possible infection, which might worsen the skin's healing response. The propensity to develop keloids may suggest a susceptibility to aberrant skin responses, even if it is not a direct cause of AK. This information may be useful in determining individual differences in AK risk.

Effects of Hormones

Skin physiology can be impacted by hormonal changes, especially during puberty, pregnancy, and menopause. Skin thickness, healing responses, and sebaceous gland activity are all influenced by hormones like testosterone and estrogen. There is, however, little direct evidence connecting the development of actinic keratosis to hormonal alterations. Hormones may have a more significant impact in circumstances that affect the skin's resilience and capacity to effectively repair UV damage.

Racial and Ethnic Components

Race and ethnicity have a major influence on the likelihood of actinic keratosis. Melanin levels are lower in people with pale skin, light-colored eyes, and red or blonde hair, which means that they have less natural protection from UV rays. On the other hand, people with darker skin tones have higher melanin levels, which provide better defense against UV-induced DNA damage and lower the risk of AK. When AKs do arise in people with darker skin, though, they might not be discovered right away and present greater health risks.

Development of Keloid and Age

Age has a crucial role in the development of actinic keratosis and keloid formation. Younger people, particularly those in their teens and twenties, have stronger collagen production during wound healing, which makes them more vulnerable to keloid formation. On the other hand, because of the cumulative effect of UV exposure over time, AKs are more common in older persons, especially those over 50. Because aging skin loses its ability to repair itself and becomes more vulnerable to cancer-causing mutations, older people are more likely to get AKs.

Additional Contributing Elements

The following additional factors raise the possibility of actinic keratosis:

1. **Immunosuppression**: People with compromised immune systems, whether as a result of HIV/AIDS or immunosuppressive drugs, are more susceptible to AK because UV-induced DNA damage is less closely monitored and repaired.

2. **Environmental Exposure**: Prolonged UV exposure from work and leisure activities, like farming, construction, and outdoor sports, greatly increases the risk of AK.

3. **Location**: Living in areas with high UV index, particularly those close to the equator or at high elevations, raises the risk of developing AK because of extended and more severe sun exposure.

4. **Lifestyle Choices**: Certain actions can worsen UV exposure and raise the risk of AK, including using tanning beds, not wearing sunscreen, and wearing insufficiently protective clothing.

5. **Preexisting Skin Conditions**: People who have continuous skin damage and healing processes, such as recurrent sunburns, photodermatoses, and certain inflammatory skin illnesses, are more susceptible to AK.

Comprehending the complex risk factors associated with actinic keratosis facilitates the development of all-encompassing preventive and therapeutic approaches, underscoring the significance of sun protection, routine skin assessments, and customized patient care tailored to individual risk profiles.

CHAPTER 3

MAKING A KELOID DIAGNOSIS

Crucial Manual for Keloids Diagnosis

Methods of Clinical Examination

The first step in diagnosing keloids is a comprehensive clinical examination. Dermatologists evaluate the scar tissue's physical attributes, such as its texture, color, size, and shape. Keloids' salient characteristics include:

- **Raised appearance:** Keloids frequently protrude beyond the skin's surface.

- **Firm consistency:** Keloids are usually firm to the touch, in contrast to hypertrophic scars.

Extension beyond original injury: One important characteristic that sets keloids apart from hypertrophic scars is their ability to extend beyond the original site of injury.

Dermatologists may also use methods like dermoscopy, which provides a thorough view of the skin's surface through the use of a specialized magnifying device. This method aids in the identification of particular vascular patterns and pigmentation changes linked to keloids.

Interviews and Patient History

Compiling a thorough medical history of the patient is essential to figuring out the causes and risk factors of keloid formation. Key points to discuss are as follows:

History of the family: There is a common genetic susceptibility to keloid formation.

Prior operations or injuries: Determining prior skin traumas that might have led to the development of keloid formation.

Symptom onset and progression: Recognising the initial appearance of the keloid and its evolution over time.

- **Previous treatments:** Recording all therapies administered and the results obtained.

- **Associated symptoms:** Ask about any discomfort, itching, or pain associated with the keloid.

A thorough interview aids in distinguishing keloids from other skin disorders and offers information on possible preventative steps to avoid recurrence in the future.

Imaging Research

Although a clinical examination is the main method used to detect keloids, imaging investigations can be helpful in certain situations:

- **Ultrasound:** High-frequency ultrasonography can assess the keloid's vascularity and depth, giving details on the degree of tissue involvement.

- **MRI:** In difficult cases where the keloid affects underlying tissues, Magnetic Resonance Imaging can be performed to evaluate deeper tissue involvement.

- **CT scans:** When keloids are linked to severe tissue distortion or functional impairment, computed tomography scans may be utilized.

A non-invasive method for determining the degree and kind of keloid scarring is imaging investigations.

Histopathology and Biopsies

If there is any uncertainty regarding the nature of the lesion, a biopsy may be carried out to confirm the diagnosis of a keloid. A typical histopathological investigation reveals:

-     **Collagen bundles:** Keloids are characterized by thick, hyalinized collagen bundles.

- **Fibroblasts:** A rise in the number of fibroblasts, the cells that produce collagen.

- **Vascularity:** Changes in blood vessel patterns from skin that are typical.

In addition, dermatofibromas, cutaneous cancers, and hypertrophic scars can be ruled out with the aid of histopathological investigation.

Distinctive Identification

It's critical to distinguish keloids from other dermatological disorders. Typical circumstances to think about are as follows:

- **Hypertrophic scars:** These do not grow past the original wound borders and may eventually recede, in contrast to keloids.

- **Dermatofibromas:** Despite having a distinct histological character, these benign skin nodules can be mistaken for keloids.

- **Cutaneous malignancies:** A biopsy is necessary to rule out certain skin cancers that manifest as elevated, nodular lesions.

Appropriate treatment planning and management are ensured by accurate differential diagnosis.

Typical Diagnostic Difficulties

The following factors make diagnosing keloids difficult:

- **Variable presentation:** The look and severity of keloids can vary widely.

Overlap with other conditions: Diagnosis might be made more difficult by similarities with hypertrophic scars and other skin abnormalities.

- **Patient history:** Inaccurate or incomplete patient history may mask risk factors and the underlying reason.

To tackle these obstacles, a methodical and comprehensive approach is needed, integrating clinical expertise with the right diagnostic instruments.

The Function of Specialists and Dermatologists

Dermatologists are essential in the diagnosis and treatment of keloids. Their knowledge is essential for:

Rough diagnosis: Distinguishing keloids from other skin disorders.

Treatment planning: Creating customized treatment schedules according to the requirements and particular state of the patient.

- **Coordination of care:** Collaborating with radiation oncologists and plastic surgeons among other experts to provide all-encompassing care.

Dermatologists also offer continuing observation and assistance to control symptoms and stop recurrence.

Technological Progress in Diagnostics

Recent technological developments have enhanced the keloid diagnosis:

- **High-resolution imaging:** Improved imaging methods make the depth and keloid structure more visible.

Molecular diagnostics: New molecular methods have made it possible to pinpoint particular genetic and biochemical indicators linked to the development of keloid formation.

- **AI and machine learning:** Based on image analysis, these technologies are being developed to help with keloids' diagnosis and distinction.

These developments raise the possibility of more accurate and customized diagnostic techniques.

Examples and Case Studies

Case studies offer important insights on keloid diagnosis and treatment. For example, consider:

- **A young woman with post-surgical keloids:** describing her course of treatment, which included adjuvant therapies and surgical excision.

- **A patient with a familial keloid tendency:** Emphasising the role of genetics and the preventative care strategy.

- **A person with numerous keloids from acne scars:** Providing an example of the difficulties and methods involved in controlling the development of widespread keloids.

These real-life examples aid in demonstrating how diagnostic concepts and treatment approaches are applied in the actual world.

Prompt Identification and Avoidance

To lessen the effects of keloids, early detection and prevention are essential. Among the strategies are:

- **Risk assessment:** Determining those who are most at risk because of a family history or a history of keloid formation.

- **Prophylactic treatments:** Applying pressure garments, silicone gels, or corticosteroid injections following trauma or surgery to stop keloid formation.

Patient education: Educating patients on the significance of taking good care of their wounds and acting quickly if any keloid symptoms manifest.

The incidence and severity of keloids can be considerably decreased by using early identification and preventative techniques that are effective.

This extensive book seeks to give readers a complete understanding of all the different facets of detecting keloids, from the most recent developments in diagnostic technology to clinical examination methods. Through the integration of comprehensive patient history, sophisticated imaging techniques, and histopathological analysis, medical practitioners can make precise diagnoses and create individualized treatment regimens.

CHAPTER 4

OPTIONS FOR TREATMENT

Topical Applications:

The initial line of defense against actinic keratoses is frequently topical therapy. The afflicted skin areas receive direct application of these drugs.

1. **Imiquimod**: This cream encourages the body's defenses against aberrant skin cells, thereby aiding in their elimination.

2. **5-Fluorouracil (5-FU)**: This drug acts by preventing the formation of aberrant skin cells, which causes them to be eliminated.

3. **Gel diclofenac sodium 3% (Solaraze)**: This gel encourages the shedding of aberrant skin cells and lessens irritation.

Injections into the Lesions:

During intralesional injections, drugs are injected straight into each unique AK lesion.

1. **5-Fluorouracil (5-FU) injections**: This technique targets particular lesions and administers the drug directly to the affected area.

Surgical Methods for Removal:

AK lesions are physically removed by surgical methods.

1. **Electrodessication and curettage**: To stop bleeding and encourage healing, the lesion is first scraped off (curettage) and then cauterized (electrodessication).

2. **Excisional surgery**: Stitches are used to seal the wound after the entire lesion is surgically removed.

Cryosurgery and Cryotherapy:

AK lesions are frozen using liquid nitrogen in cryotherapy.

1. **Liquid nitrogen cryotherapy**: The aberrant cells are frozen and then slough off as the skin heals.

Laser Treatment:

Laser therapy targets and destroys AK lesions with concentrated light radiation.

1. **CO2 laser**: The top layers of skin that contain AK cells are vaporized by this laser.

Radiation Treatment:

High-energy radiation is used in radiation treatment to destroy AK cells.

1. **X-ray radiation**: AK lesions are treated with targeted radiation beams.

Silicone gel sheets and pressure:

These techniques are frequently used to enhance the appearance of scars after therapy.

1. **Pressure therapy**: You can lessen scarring by applying pressure to the area that has healed.

2. **Silica gel sheets**: To flatten and fade scars, apply these sheets over healed wounds.

Home and Alternative Remedies:

Some people advise alternative therapies that aren't as clinically proven.

1. When applied topically, **apple cider vinegar** is thought to aid in the removal of AK lesions.

2. **Aloe vera**: This plant's gel is said to offer calming and restorative qualities.

Combinatorial Therapies:

In many cases, combining various therapy approaches can lead to better results.

1. **Topical and surgical**: For lesions that are resistant to topical treatment, surgical removal is the next step.

2. **Laser and cryotherapy**: For thorough lesion eradication, combine laser therapy and cryotherapy.

Assessing the Success of Treatment:

Evaluation of therapy outcomes is essential after completion.

1. **Clinical examination**: The physician looks for indications of healing or recurrence in the treated area.

2. **Biopsy**: To look for any remaining aberrant cells, a biopsy may be performed in specific circumstances.

3. **Feedback from patients**: Patients should let their healthcare practitioner know about any changes or worries.

Every treatment choice offers advantages and things to think about. The amount of lesions, where they are located, and your general health will all be taken into consideration by your dermatologist to identify the best course of action. It's critical to do routine follow-ups to track advancement and handle any fresh issues.

CHAPTER 5

PREVENTIVE TECHNIQUES

Value of Prompt Intervention

Effective management of actinic keratosis (AK) requires early intervention. Early identification and intervention can stop AK from worsening and leading to more serious skin diseases such as squamous cell carcinoma. It lowers the possibility of problems, boosts the results of treatment, and improves the patient's prognosis overall.

Adequate Methods for Treating Wounds

Using the right wound care techniques after treatment is crucial to accelerating healing and lowering the risk of infection. This entails cleaning the afflicted area, applying topical drugs or dressings as directed, and carefully adhering to prescription directions from the healthcare professional. Taking good care of wounds can also reduce pain and scarring while the wound heals.

Preventing Skin Injury

Activities that could aggravate or traumatize the skin should be avoided by patients, particularly in places where AK has been treated. This includes avoiding harsh chemicals or abrasive materials, shielding the skin from prolonged sun exposure, and being aware of any clothing or accessories that can rub against areas that have had treatment.

The function of gels and silicone sheets

After AK therapy, silicone sheets and gels are frequently advised for scar control. They lessen redness and irritation, smooth out and soften scars, and enhance the appearance of skin overall. Consistent application of silicone products can improve the aesthetic results of AK treatment.

The Usage of Pressure Garments

Pressure garments could be suggested in some circumstances to control scarring or encourage wound healing following AK treatment. These clothes gently press against the skin, which can promote tissue healing, increase blood flow, and lessen edema. For best effects, wearers must adhere to wearing schedules and ensure proper fitting.

Medications for Prevention

In individuals with multiple or recurring AK lesions, certain drugs, such as topical creams or gels containing imiquimod, fluorouracil, or diclofenac, may be recommended for preventative purposes. These drugs help stop the growth of new AK lesions, lessen inflammation, and target aberrant skin cells.

Changes to Lifestyle

Promoting lifestyle changes is crucial for the prevention of AK. This entails taking sun safety precautions including wearing protective clothes, applying sunscreen frequently, looking for shade during the hottest parts of the day, and staying away from tanning beds and sunlamps. Skin health is also influenced by healthy lifestyle choices such as abstaining from smoking and eating a balanced diet.

Continuous Monitoring and Follow-Up

Patients should see their doctor for follow-up appointments regularly to assess any new lesions, discuss any concerns or consequences, and track the effectiveness of AK treatment. Regular skin examinations are essential for spotting early indications of skin cancer and guaranteeing prompt treatment.

Awareness and Education of Patients

It is crucial to inform patients about AK, its risk factors, preventative measures, and the value of early detection. More informed patients are better able to take charge of their skin health, seek prompt medical attention, and follow treatment and preventive guidelines.

Progress in Preventive Medicine

Promising developments and ongoing research are being made in AK prevention tactics. To improve efficacy, lessen adverse effects, and increase treatment options for individuals with AK, novel topical medicines, photodynamic therapy approaches, and immunotherapy options are being developed.

Together, these preventive techniques offer a whole approach to controlling actinic keratosis, highlighting the significance of prompt intervention, appropriate wound care, lifestyle adjustments, and continuous patient education and awareness.

CHAPTER 6

COEXISTING WITH KELOIDS

Effects on Emotion and Psychology

Living with Keloids can have a major impact on a person's mental and emotional health. People can feel a variety of things, such as humiliation, frustration, and self-consciousness. The obvious form of keloids can cause social anxiety and negatively impact an individual's quality of life, particularly when they arise on prominent places like the hands, neck, or face. Those who believe that keloids have a major impact on their look are more likely to experience depression and anxiety. It's critical to acknowledge these emotional effects and seek the proper mental health care, such as therapy or counseling, to deal with these emotions.

Coping Mechanisms and Support Networks

Creating efficient coping mechanisms is crucial to controlling the psychological and emotional strain brought on by keloids. These tactics could consist of:

- **Acceptance and Self-Compassion:** Developing self-compassion and learning to accept oneself as one looks can help lessen unpleasant emotions.

- **Support Groups:** Participating in live or virtual support groups helps foster a feeling of camaraderie and comprehension. It might be empowering to share experiences with those who suffer from comparable conditions.

- **Professional Assistance:** Consulting with mental health specialists, such as psychologists or counselors, can offer coping mechanisms for handling the emotional load.

Skincare Protocols for Skin Prone to Keratosis

For people who are prone to keloids, proper skin care is essential for managing pre-existing scars and preventing additional skin trauma:

- **Gentle Cleaning:** Prevent inflammation by using gentle, non-irritating cleaners.

- **Moisturization:** Applying moisturizer regularly can help keep the skin's barrier intact and guard against dryness and cracking.

- **Sun Protection:** Using broad-spectrum sunscreen to shield the skin from the sun can help prevent keloids from becoming hyperpigmented.

- **Preventing Trauma:** Reduce any behaviors or actions that may lead to cuts on the skin, like picking at the skin or wearing tight clothing.

Tips for Concealment and Makeup

Concealing keloids with makeup can increase self-esteem and confidence:

- **Colour Correctors:** Green primers help counteract keloids' redness.

- **High-Coverage Foundations:** To integrate the keloid with the surrounding skin, use foundations with strong coverage.

- **Setting Products:** To guarantee that makeup stays in place all day, use setting spray or powder.

Outfit Selection and Comfort

The way that keloids look and feel can be greatly influenced by clothing:

- **Soft Fabrics:** To lessen irritation, wear soft, breathable clothing.

- **Loose-Fitting Clothing:** To prevent pressure and friction on keloids, wear clothing that fits loosely.

- **Strategic Fashion Choices:** If you feel more at ease wearing items that cover your keloids, go for long sleeves or scarves.

Social and Career Difficulties

Keloids may provide particular social and occupational difficulties, such as:

Workplace Accommodations: If adjustments, such as lenient dress codes, are required, be upfront with employers about your illness.

- **Social Interactions:** Be ready with answers to questions on your keloids so you can confidently navigate social settings.

-   **Professional Help:** To navigate professional contexts with keloids, think about consulting mentors or career counselors.

Body Image and Self-Esteem

Body image and self-esteem can be severely impacted by keloids:

- **Positive Affirmations:** To increase self-esteem, repeat affirmations to yourself.

- **Body Positivity:** Join groups and initiatives that promote body positivity to build a network of people who will support you.

- **Therapeutic Support:** Counselling can assist in addressing problems related to body image and cultivating a more positive self-image.

Using Resources and Support Groups

Getting the correct help can have a profound impact:

- **Online Communities:** Reddit and other websites, as well as certain Facebook groups, can provide guidance and assistance.

- **Local Support Groups:** Check with community centers or hospitals to find local support groups.

Expert Associations: Associations like the American Academy of Dermatology provide information and assistance to those with skin disorders.

Motivational Tales of Triumphing Against Keloids

Perusing accounts from individuals who have effectively tackled their keloids can be immensely inspiring:

- **Personal Blogs:** A lot of people share their experiences online, offering wisdom and motivation.

- **Films and Articles:** Seek out films or articles that highlight individual accounts of perseverance and triumph over hardship.

- **Social Media Influencers:** To learn how others manage their everyday lives, follow influencers who candidly share their experiences with keloids.

Extended-Term Management Schemes

It's vital to manage keloids over the long term:

- **Regular Visits with the Dermatologist:** Continue with routine examinations to monitor and treat keloids as necessary.

- **Personalised Treatment Plans:** Create a customized treatment plan in collaboration with medical professionals. This plan may involve topical medications, injections, or laser therapy.

- **Healthy Lifestyle:** To support general skin health, maintain a healthy lifestyle that includes frequent exercise and a balanced diet.

Maintain Mental Health: Constantly partake in practices like mindfulness, meditation, and counseling that enhance mental health.

People with keloids can create a complete plan for controlling their disease and enhancing their quality of life by taking care of each of these factors.

CHAPTER 7

INVESTIGATIONS AND PROGRESS

Notable Achievers in Keloid Science

The study of keloid scars has a long history, going back to ancient civilizations when records of scars resembling keloid were discovered. However, the first recorded medical descriptions of keloids date back to the 19th century, marking the beginning of current scientific inquiry into keloids. The mid-20th century elucidation of keloid pathophysiology was a key milestone as it redirected attention toward understanding the involvement of inflammation, fibroblasts, and collagen in keloid formation.

Recent Trends in Research

Multidisciplinary studies in tissue engineering, immunology, genetics, and dermatology are being conducted on keloids nowadays. examining the molecular mechanisms behind keloid formation, examining immunomodulatory treatments, and employing cutting-edge imaging methods to describe the composition and shape of keloid formation are among the current trends.

Innovative Therapies and Treatments

Advancements in the management of keloid formation have been observed in recent times, encompassing the creation of specific biological medicines such as growth factor inhibitors and anti-inflammatory cytokines. By treating the underlying causes and symptoms of keloid formation, innovations such as silicone gel sheets, cryotherapy, and microneedling have also improved outcomes.

Genetics's Role in Keloid Research

Keloid susceptibility is mostly determined by genetic predisposition, and current research attempts to pinpoint particular genetic markers linked to keloid formation. Personalized therapy has been made possible by the unraveling of the complex genetic architecture of keloids by genome-wide association studies (GWAS) made possible by advances in genomic sequencing and bioinformatics.

Advances in Pharmacology

Novel medications targeting TGF-β signaling, matrix metalloproteinases (MMPs), and inflammatory mediators—three important pathways implicated in keloid pathogenesis—have been developed as a result of pharmacological study. To control keloids, topical, intralesional, and systemic pharmacotherapies are being optimized for safety and efficacy.

Recent Advances in Surgery

Novel surgical techniques including laser-assisted keloidectomy, tension-reducing methods, and modified W-plasty have reduced recurrence rates and increased surgical success. For comprehensive keloid management, combining surgery with adjuvant medications such as radiation or intralesional corticosteroids is a viable approach.

Photo- and Laser-Assisted Therapies

Keloid treatment has been transformed by advances in laser technology, such as intense pulsed light (IPL) devices, fractional lasers, and pulsed dye lasers (PDL). With fewer adverse effects and a decreased scar volume, these techniques address the vascular and collagen components of keloids.

Examining Alternative Treatments

Alternative remedies for keloids are being researched using a variety of techniques, including extracorporeal shock wave therapy (ESWT), vitamin-based therapies, photodynamic therapy (PDT), and herbal extracts. These methods provide complementary choices, especially for individuals who prefer non-invasive therapies or have contraindications.

Cooperative Research Initiatives

Research and therapy for keloid disorders have advanced faster thanks to collaboration between industrial partners, scientists, and physicians. Collaboration is facilitated by worldwide consortiums, common databases, and multicenter clinical trials. This allows for data sharing, protocol standardization, and validation of novel treatments.

Advances in the Future and New Therapies

With new treatments like targeted gene editing, tissue-engineered constructions or stem cells for regenerative medicine, and immunotherapy-based methods, the field of keloid research has a bright future. It is expected that precision medicine approaches customized to each patient's genetic profile and scar properties will completely change the way that keloid treatment is approached.

This thorough summary captures the ever-changing field of keloid research, emphasizing its historical roots, present developments, and potential future directions for better comprehension and treatment of this difficult dermatological ailment.

CHAPTER 8

SOCIETAL AND CULTURAL VIEWPOINTS

Keloids in Various Societies

Definition and Significance in Culture:

Overgrown scars that grow outside of the original location of injury are called keloids. Their importance differs depending on the culture:

African Cultures: Traditional scarification techniques can be used to purposefully generate keloids, which are frequently seen as a symbol of power and beauty.

- **Asian Cultures:** Keloids are frequently seen negatively in various Asian communities, where they are thought to be an indication of inadequate recovery.

- **Western Cultures:** Generally considered a medical condition that has to be treated or a cosmetic concern.

Customs and Traditions:

- **Scarification:** Intentional keloid creation through scarification is a rite of passage for some African cultures.

- **Tattooing and Piercing:** Different cultures have varying views on these bodily alterations, and keloids can arise from tattoos or piercings.

Historical Perceptions of Keloids

Sensible Opinions:

- **Egyptian Medicine:** Treatments for keloids and other aberrant scars are described in early Egyptian medical books.

- **Greek and Roman Periods:** Documentary evidence points to a combination of medical intervention attempts and acceptance.

From the Mediaeval to the Modern Era:

- **Mediaeval Europe:** Keloids were sometimes misinterpreted and connected to moral or spiritual transgressions.

19th and 20th Centuries: As medical research advanced, keloids were examined more thoroughly, which resulted in a move away from cultural interpretation and towards medical therapy.

Misconceptions and Stigma in Society

Misunderstanding Prevalence:

Aesthetic Concerns: Rather than being a medical disease, keloids are frequently thought of as only cosmetic flaws.

Myths About Contagion: A few cultures have the false belief that keloids are communicable.

Sigma's Effect:

- **Self-Esteem Issues:** Because of cultural beauty standards, people with keloids may experience low self-esteem.

- **Social Isolation:** Social disengagement and mental health issues can result from a fear of being judged.

Keloids in Media and Literature

Literary Representation:

- **Symbolism:** Keloids can represent several topics, including identity, resiliency, and trauma.

- **Characterization:** Keloids can be used by writers to illustrate a character's cultural background or personal issues, giving them more depth.

Shown in the Media:

- **Positive Representation:** Media portrayals of keloids are becoming more positive, with an emphasis on variety and acceptance.

Negative Stereotypes: Keloids are still sometimes used to represent villains or misfits, which perpetuates unfavorable perceptions.

Testimonials and Personal Narratives

Stories:

- **Resilience and Acceptance:** A lot of people relate their experiences of accepting their keloids, which creates a feeling of solidarity and community.

-    **Difficulties Overcame:** Individual narratives frequently emphasize the psychological and physical suffering connected to keloids, along with the path towards locating a suitable remedy.

Affect on Lobbying:

Awareness Campaigns: An important aspect of advocacy is the use of personal narratives to humanize the issue and raise awareness.

Culture's Influence on Treatment Decisions

Modern vs. Conventional Treatments:

- **Herbal Remedies:** Certain societies value traditional herbal remedies over contemporary medical care.

- **Medical Treatments:** Depending on their culture's acceptance of medical technology, some may prefer laser therapy, corticosteroid injections, or surgical removal.

Cultural Belief Influence:

- **Spiritual Healing:** Some cultures treat keloids using holistic or spiritual methods that combine medical procedures with cultural beliefs.

Campaigns for Advocacy and Awareness

Aims for the Campaign:

- **Education:** Raising public awareness about keloids to lessen stigma and foster compassion.

- **Support Networks:** Forming support groups for keloid victims.

Notable Initiatives:

- **International Initiatives:** To promote awareness and provide funding for research, groups like the International Keloid Research Foundation operate on a global scale.

Local Efforts: To optimize impact, community-based campaigns customize their initiatives to local cultural circumstances.

Dealing with Bias and Discrimination

Social Bias and the Workplace:

- **Employment Discrimination:** Hiring processes may be biased against people who have visible keloids.

- **Social Prejudice:** Keloids have the potential to cause social prejudice, which can harm interpersonal relationships and interactions.

Methods for Resolving Bias:

* **Policy Changes:** Pushing for anti-discrimination laws in schools and workplaces.

- **Public Education:** Introducing campaigns to dispel prejudice and inform the public about the medical significance of keloids.

Treatment with Cultural Sensitivity

The Significance of Sensitivity

- **Respecting Beliefs:** When recommending therapies, healthcare professionals must take into account cultural beliefs and customs.

- **Inclusive Care:** Creating treatment programs that take cultural preferences into account and offer care that is competent in various cultures.

Optimal Techniques:

- **Patient Education:** Educating patients about all possible options for care while taking into consideration their cultural background.

- **Collaborative Approach:** When appropriate, collaborating with traditional healers and cultural leaders to incorporate modern and traditional techniques.

International Views on Keloid Control

Local Strategies:

- **Africa:** Integrating contemporary medical procedures with customary methods.

Asia: Stressing cutting-edge medical interventions along with an increasing understanding of keloid-specific concerns.

Western Countries: Concentrating on advocacy and support networks in addition to research and therapy development.

Global Difficulties:

Accessibility: Guaranteeing treatment that is both inexpensive and effective for everyone, anywhere.

- **Cultural Barriers:** Dispelling cultural prejudices and misconceptions via international advocacy and education initiatives.

By taking into account these diverse viewpoints, we may promote a more accepting and compassionate approach to keloid management, improving the prognosis for patients as well as their quality of life.

CHAPTER 9

YOUNGER KELOIDS

Rate Among Kids and Teenagers

Overgrowths of scar tissue that grow outside of the initial wound borders are called keloids. Keloids are very uncommon in children and adolescents, although their prevalence varies greatly in comparison to adults. However, in this age group, keloid formation may be more likely due to certain factors like genetic predisposition, skin type, and type of skin damage (such as surgical scars or ear piercings). Research indicates that keloids are more common in those with darker complexion, with higher rates seen in Asian, African, and Hispanic populations.

Particular Difficulties with Paediatric Patients

When it comes to keloids, pediatric patients have special difficulties. Their skin is still growing, which may have an impact on how well they heal and react to medical interventions. Furthermore, the emergence of keloids may cause youngsters to suffer from more severe psychological anguish, which can negatively impact their social connections and sense of self. Because skin grows dynamically, keloids can also alter in size and shape over time, sometimes requiring continuous therapy changes and maintenance.

Treatment Issues to Be Aware of with Young Patients

A careful balance between minimizing potential side effects and maximizing efficacy is needed when treating keloids in children. Conventional treatments include:

- **Topical treatments:** Corticosteroid creams and silicone gel sheets can help flatten keloids and lessen associated discomfort.

- **Intralesional corticosteroid injections:** Although they can lessen swelling and the extent of keloid formation, these injections may hurt younger people.

- **Cryotherapy:** Using liquid nitrogen to freeze the keloid; frequently used in conjunction with other therapies.

- **Laser therapy:** May help reduce the appearance of keloids by flattening them.

Surgical excision: Usually explored in cases where non-surgical therapies are ineffective, but a keloid recurrence is possible.

The location and size of the keloid, together with the patient's age and general condition, all influence the therapy option. It is frequently required to use a multidisciplinary strategy that includes dermatologists, pediatricians, and occasionally plastic surgeons.

Children's Psychological Effects

Keloids can have a significant psychological effect on kids. Visible keloids can cause social anxiety, bullying, and self-consciousness, especially if they are on the hands, neck, or face. Teenagers may be especially at risk because of their increased self-awareness during puberty. It is imperative to address these psychological components; consulting with mental health specialists or counselors can help kids get the help they need to deal with the emotional difficulties of having keloids.

Guidance for Parents and Carers

The management of pediatric keloids is greatly dependent on parents and carers. They ought to be informed about the causes of keloids, available treatments, and the significance of following a prescribed course of action. Parents' emotional support can lessen the psychological toll on their kids. Carers should also be aware of possible keloid formation triggers, such as injuries or ear piercings, and seek early intervention if a keloid begins to develop.

Strategies for Early Intervention

Effective management of pediatric keloids requires early intervention. Proactive measures, like the following, should be done as soon as a child sustains a wound or skin injury to avoid keloid formation:

- Protecting and cleaning the wound.

- Applying pressure garments or silicone gel sheets as directed.

- Using topical medications as prescribed by a medical professional.

- Quickly seeking medical advice and keeping an eye out for any abnormal scar growth at the wound site.

Keloids can be treated early to stop them from getting bigger and more difficult to treat.

Children's Preventive Measures

For kids who have a recognized risk of developing keloids, prevention is key. These include:

- Avoiding needless skin harm, such as elective piercings or tattoos.

- Using pressure earrings after ear piercings to decrease keloid risk.

- Applying sunscreen to scars to prevent darkening and worsening of keloids.

- Ensuring good wound care and hygiene.

Teaching kids about these steps can encourage them to actively participate in maintaining the health of their skin.

Success Stories and Case Studies

Success stories and case studies can provide hope and direction for families suffering from pediatric keloids. For instance, one case study might detail a youngster who effectively controlled keloids using a combination of intralesional corticosteroids and laser therapy, leading to considerable improvement. Another narrative can emphasize an adolescent who overcomes the psychological burden of keloids with the help of a supportive school environment and counseling. These accounts can highlight the varied spectrum of treatment outcomes and coping mechanisms.

Research on Pediatric Keloids

Ongoing research is necessary to better the understanding and management of pediatric keloids. Current studies are studying the genetic variables that lead to keloid formation, the efficacy of novel treatments such as biologic medicines, and the long-term consequences of various therapeutic techniques. Additionally, research is concentrating on the creation of more effective and minimally invasive treatment alternatives designed especially for kids and teenagers.

Long-Term Outlook for Pediatric Patients

The prognosis for children with keloids varies over time. While some children may improve on their own over time, others might need constant care to reduce symptoms and avoid recurrence. Results can be considerably improved by adequate and timely intervention. Despite the difficulties caused by keloids, many youngsters can anticipate leading normal, healthy lives with advancements in therapy and a greater understanding of the problem.

Pediatric patients with keloids face particular difficulties that call for particular attention and treatment. A thorough strategy is necessary, encompassing everything from early intervention and therapy to psychological support and preventive measures. The greatest outcomes and a good quality of life are guaranteed for children with keloids because of ongoing research and success stories that give hope and direction.

CHAPTER 10

SOURCES & ADDITIONAL READING

Extensive Terminology Dictionary

1. **Keloid**: An excessive development of scar tissue surrounding an injury or wound.

2. **Hypertrophic Scar**: An elevated scar that remains contained within the initial wound's bounds.

3. **Collagen**: A protein found in skin and other connective tissues that is vital to the healing of wounds.

4. **Fibroblast**: Collagen-producing cells essential to the healing of wounds.

5. **Silicone Gel Sheeting**: A direct application to the skin that treats keloids without intrusions.

6. **Injections of Corticosteroid**: Anti-inflammatory shots intended to lessen the size and symptoms of keloid formation.

7. **Surgical Excision**: The removal of keloids surgically, frequently with further therapies to avoid recurrence.

8. **Radiotherapy**: Following surgical excision, radiation therapy is utilized to prevent keloid recurrence.

9. **Cryotherapy**: Freezing treatment that eliminates extra tissue in the treatment of keloids.

10. **Interferon Therapy**: Interferon proteins are used in treatment to shrink keloid size and stop recurrence.

Important Groups and Associations

1. **American Academy of Dermatology (AAD)**: Offers reference materials and keloids information.

2. The American Society for Dermatologic Surgery (ASDS) provides information on available treatments for keloids.

3. Guidelines and assistance for plastic surgeons treating keloids are provided by the **American Society of Plastic Surgeons (ASPS)**.

4. **International Society of Dermatology (ISD)**: Addresses keloids and other international dermatological concerns.

5. **Keloid Support Group**: Local and virtual support groups that provide emotional support and a platform for people to share their stories for those impacted by keloids.

Suggested Readings and Articles

1. "Keloids: Pathogenesis, Clinical Features, and Management" is an extensive book that discusses the causes of keloid formation and available treatments.

2. A patient-friendly resource outlining keloids and their therapies is **"Understanding Keloids: A Guide for Patients and Healthcare Providers"**.

3. **American Academy of Dermatology Journal**: Disseminates information on keloids, including research results and recommendations for therapy.

4. An academic study addressing the most recent developments in keloid research and therapy is **" Keloids Uncovered: A Comprehensive Review of Pathophysiology to Treatment Strategies"**.

Online Communities and Resources

1. **Keloid Forum**: A discussion forum for keloid experiences, care, and assistance.

2. **Keloid Awareness Website**: offers patient tales, treatment choices, and information on keloids.

3. **Keloid Research Hub**: Provides information related to keloid studies for researchers and medical professionals.

4. **Keloid Support Groups on Social Media**: Twitter hashtags, Reddit forums, and Facebook groups devoted to keloid support and awareness.

Journals and Research Databases

1. **PubMed**: A resource containing in-depth research papers on keloids and associated subjects.

2. **Google Scholar**: Offers access to academic books, research papers, and articles on keloids.

3. **Journal of Dermatological Science**: Disseminates studies on the etiology of keloid pathogenesis, therapeutic response, and innovative treatments.

4. **Dermatology Online Journal**: Offers case studies and papers about research and management of keloid formation.

Conferences and Professional Associations

1. **American Association of Plastic Surgeons (AAPS)**: Organises seminars and conferences on the latest developments in keloid treatment.

2. **International Society of Plastic and Aesthetic Surgeons (ISPAS)**: This organization focuses on innovations in plastic surgery, such as the management of keloids.

3. **World Congress of Dermatology (WCD)**: Workshops and sessions on scar management and keloids will be held.

Advocacy Groups for Patients

1. **Keloid Awareness Foundation**: Promotes treatment access, education, and patient rights for keloid patients.

2. **Global Skin Foundation**: Promotes awareness and advocacy for skin health issues, such as keloids.

Public Sector and Non-Profit Establishments

1. **National Institutes of Health (NIH)**: Provides funding for studies on treatment modalities and keloids.

2. **World Health Organisation (WHO)**: Addresses issues related to global health, such as keloids and other skin diseases.

3. **American Skin Association (ASA)**: Promotes skin problems and funds research on keloid lesions.

Instructional Resources and Manuals

1. **Keloid Treatment Brochures**: These provide information on treatment options and expectations and can be found online and at dermatological clinics.

2. **Patient Education Videos**: Made available by medical professionals to inform patients about keloids and how to handle them.

3. **Keloid Prevention Tips**: Instructional resources emphasizing methods to stop the production of keloid scars following surgeries or injuries.

How to Keep Up with Research on Keloid

1. **Subscribe to Medical Journals**: Keep an eye out for fresh keloid research by regularly reading publications like Dermatology, Journal of Investigative Dermatology, and Dermatologic Surgery.

2. **Follow Professional Organisations**: Keep up with webinars, conferences, and newsletters from AAD, ASDS, and ASPS, among other organizations.

3. **Connect with Research Institutions**: Get the latest information from academic institutions and research centers working on keloids.

4. **Join Online Forums**: To keep up to date on the newest therapies and scientific discoveries, participate in conversations in keloid forums and social media groups.

Through the use of this thorough guide and resources, advocates, medical professionals, researchers, and people impacted by keloids can all have a better understanding of, ability to oversee, and support keloid-related activities and treatments.